The Beautician

Mary M.

ISBN 978-1-716-40993-6

The Beautician

by

Mary M.

A practice guide in 12 lessons

to become a real Beautician

Introduction

This booklet, which holds 12 lessons, is designed for people who want to approach cosmetics, for themselves, or for their families, or who have the intention to make it their profession without loosing time and money. But it is also designed for many others, so that they could know human body in this side. This marvellous machine, that still we always know too little. The readers deserve a certificate for their interest: I believe that young people could become keen and for this they deserve an award.

Preface

Read carefully each lesson, because each word is meaningful for it is the substance of vast concepts summarized in short with the aim to be assimilated better and in a short time.

Each lesson is preceded by a list of materials and tools needed. To get the professional tools or to have advices you can refer to a specialized shop.

Mary is willing to help those needing more informations and hints on the covered subjects, or wanting a visage reading for the most appropriate make up and hair style: you just need to write to the address indicated below and get in touch.

It is possible to ask for the conferment of the course attendance's certificate: to know the issue procedure, send to the e-mail address below the answers to the verification questions that follow the lessons.

ringthebell@libero.it

What is needed in this lesson:

- A beautician armchair with headrest
- A cloth mantle
- A headband to free the face from hair
- A wall mirror

The beautician
Introduction and analysis

Dear student, it is now starting the accelerated course of cosmetics and I, your direct teacher, wish from you all your faith and intelligence or at least goodwill, that goodwill which gives certainty of a good result.

Break down uncertainty and discouragement: you have to know that I will guide you time after time with my skills and experience to let you obtain the best results in becoming a good beautician.
In this first introductory lesson, I will show some essential tricks and rules, and some practical and historic notions as well.

The rules are:
The BEAUTICIAN shall accept this work with reliability because this way he will be trustworthy for whose who rely on him. He must always have clean gown and look, and hands also before and after each treatment with well finished finger-nails. Also all the tools

used in the treatments must be washed before and after with water and soap or better sterilized.

The workplace must be calm, discreet or with a background music: that will help the client to relax the muscles, obtaining this way a better result. It is important to work on healthy skins; this is to avoid reddening and complications. Only in the case of *seborrhoeic* skins, or with *acne*, they can be cured with specific products for these specific case.

The client must be guided, advised, aiming always to the good result of the treatment, in fact that is what the client expects: to improve her aesthetic appearance, because since ever woman love to primp, to take care of herself, to be beautiful.
Let's remember the past: the French women were the first to launch the trend of blonde hair and to be imitated by the women of all the world who lightened the hair with plant leaves and with any other empirical method.
Also the history of ancient Egypt reminds us how much its women cared of their beauty and their jet-black hair. Or also Poppaea as told in the movie on Nero, how much she cared of her skin at the point to take baths in donkey mare milk, which is rich in emollient proprieties. Also into the ancient Roman tombs there were found many small jars containing creams and various ointments that they jealously kept hidden; all of this should make us to ponder and understand that woman needs us, because we give her our trustworthiness and professionalism.

Analysis of the visage

We invite the client to seat with a mantle on the shoulders and with a headband around the face to free it from hair and we look it carefully through the mirror to notice if it is:

- round, square, oval, oblong or triangular;
- the lips are thin or full;
- the eyes little, big, close, distant, bulging or regular;
- the forehead high or low;
- and if the height is tall or short.

Examine with few glances the type and the work to be done.

Now, rest the client's head against the armchair, placing you at its right; examine the skin, touching it with the right hand along the *seborrhoeic* line which runs along forehead nose chin and determine this way the kind of skin to be worked.

If in these points above you notice that the skin is *oily*, with dilated pores, then it needs de-oiling and astringent products; if on the contrary it is *dry* it needs to be nourished.

If it is *soft* at the touch, it needs normal products or for mixed skins.

End of first lesson

Verification questions:

- Where is it the seborrhoeic line?
- In the past, who launched the blonde trend?
- Who in ancient Rome was taking baths in donkey milk?
- What ancient Egypt's women loved most to take care of?

What is needed in this lesson:

- A cloth triangle
- Two small beautician sponges
- A cleansing milk or cream
- Water
- Paper wipes
- A towel for the face
- A distilled water vaporizer
- A terry cloth
- A blackheads removal tool
- Rose water

The Skin and its cleansing

The skin covers the human body and it is large nearly 2 m².

It is composed of several layers, which we could resume in three of mayor importance: the epidermis, which is the one that can be touched and where the horny layer forms, with its dead cells, ready to be removed to make room for the new born.

Derma and hypoderma, are the most important layers, where all the glands, vessels and hair are born.

The hypoderma contains also the fat layer that works as a support in case of illnesses or prolonged slimming diets, to which it

compensates as a reserve of energies, and even as insulator because works as a cushion in case of tumbles and contusions.
The epidermis is in tight relation with the other layers inside, hence the skin pores are vehicles for the metabolism.

To clean the skin, remove the dead cells, (small cuticles that we can sometimes see to fall by themselves), is the primary and indispensable thing to do, because not only we will obtain a more luminous skin, but we will make easier the metabolism for a good body functioning.

Cleansing (demaquillage)

After having freed the face from hair, with a cloth triangle tied behind the nape, take a small sponge wet with some cleansing milk: rub it on the eyes and remove the make up and impurities, then on the lips, if there is lipstick, and lastly clean neck and face, starting from low to high removing any impurity; repeat with cleaned sponge, a second time.

Vaporizer

Each time that it happens a neglected and opaque skin, which needs a careful cleansing, it is good to have some vaporization.

Put a litre of distilled water into the vaporizer, turn it on, and as soon as the vapour comes out, place it in front of the client's face (preventing burns) for five minutes: the skin this way will be sprinkled and clean deeply. If you do not have a professional vaporizer, you can get a vapour just the same with a homely way with a simple pot of boiling water (as for suffumigations).

We could also remove, if it is the case, the blackheads (little black spots) or the whiteheads (little grains in the skin of keratotic origin).

This operation is performed with the blackheads remover, a small metal tool like a spire of wire, which is handled pushing, in the point of the blackhead to excise it, helping oneself with the other hand by stretching the skin.

After this operation run over the face a cloth wet with rose or cool water.

End of second lesson

Verification questions:

- How many layers does skin have?
- What demaquillage means?
- Where are born the glands, the vessels, the hair?
- When the vaporization have to be done?

What is needed in this lesson:

- A gel cream demaquillante
- A little sponge
- Water
- Paper wipes

The descaling

In this lesson we will talk about the descaling, yet pondering the word the meaning is clear: in fact to descale means to clean deeply the surface of the skin, to which weather, sun, grease and dust have hardened till the point to need a methodical removal.

It may be as the surface of a furniture, the inside of a vase and so on, but we will deal with the skin of the face.

The descaling is executed after the demaquillage, when the skin appear to be very neglected and hardened having not received due care for much time. It is thus needing a renewal of the dead cells which, laid on the surface, have created a barrier for the metabolism, forming a horny layer.

The descaling is done applying a gel cream demaquillante rubbing and caressing with a circular movement, using the thumb, the index and the middle fingers of both hands.

Execution

After having applied the cream on the face, with both hands and standing behind the client, execute the true treatment:
pass the index and middle fingers of both hands around the orbicular of the lips, starting from the mouth centre up to the edges; stop there and with only the thumbs press with a small circular movement to close the movement (see illustration 4 page 21). Repeat three times.

Now restarting from the mouth centre repeat continuing up to the ears, stop there and press with the thumbs with the usual small movement in circle to close the movement, and repeat three times.

Now start from the nostrils with circular movement and continue up to the nose base between the brows and on the forehead to then return on the mouth edges and go up again up to the ears making the usual small circle.

Then restart with the two hands from the chin and with medium and index of both hands, in front: press the skin between the fingers, with small pinches, on all the mouth line up to the nose on both sides of the mouth; then pass with a caressing movement, alternating these two movement four times.

Now with the thumbs of both hands, which will stay closed as a fist, make many small circles starting from the chin, ears, mouth, nose, cheeks, eyes, and forehead.

Then with both opened hands start from the lower part of the neck and up for all the face up to the forehead with a "kneading" movement, as to amalgamate all the stages of the massage.

Then with a damp small beautician sponge, remove the cream with rotatory movements, taking altogether the dead cells with it.

Memorize well these massage movements, so precious also for the anti-age massage, with nourishing creams and oils.

End of third lesson

Verification questions:

- What's the use of descaling?
- Where dead cells are laid?
- What cream is used for descaling?
- What are the movements for descaling?

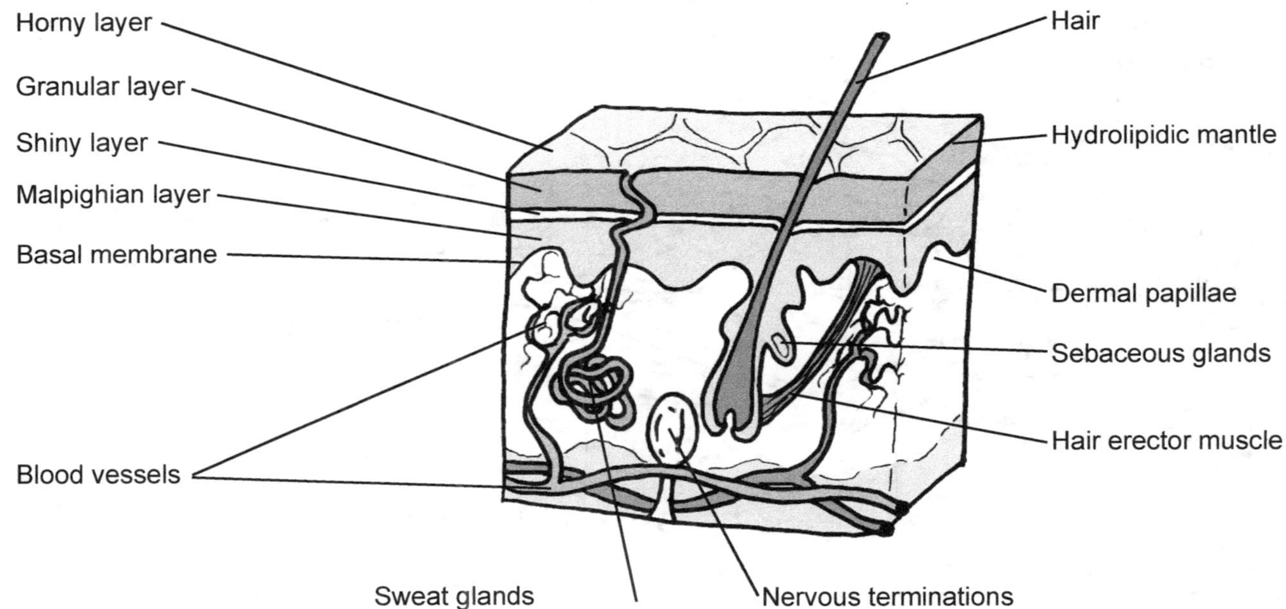

Illustration 1 - Skin structure

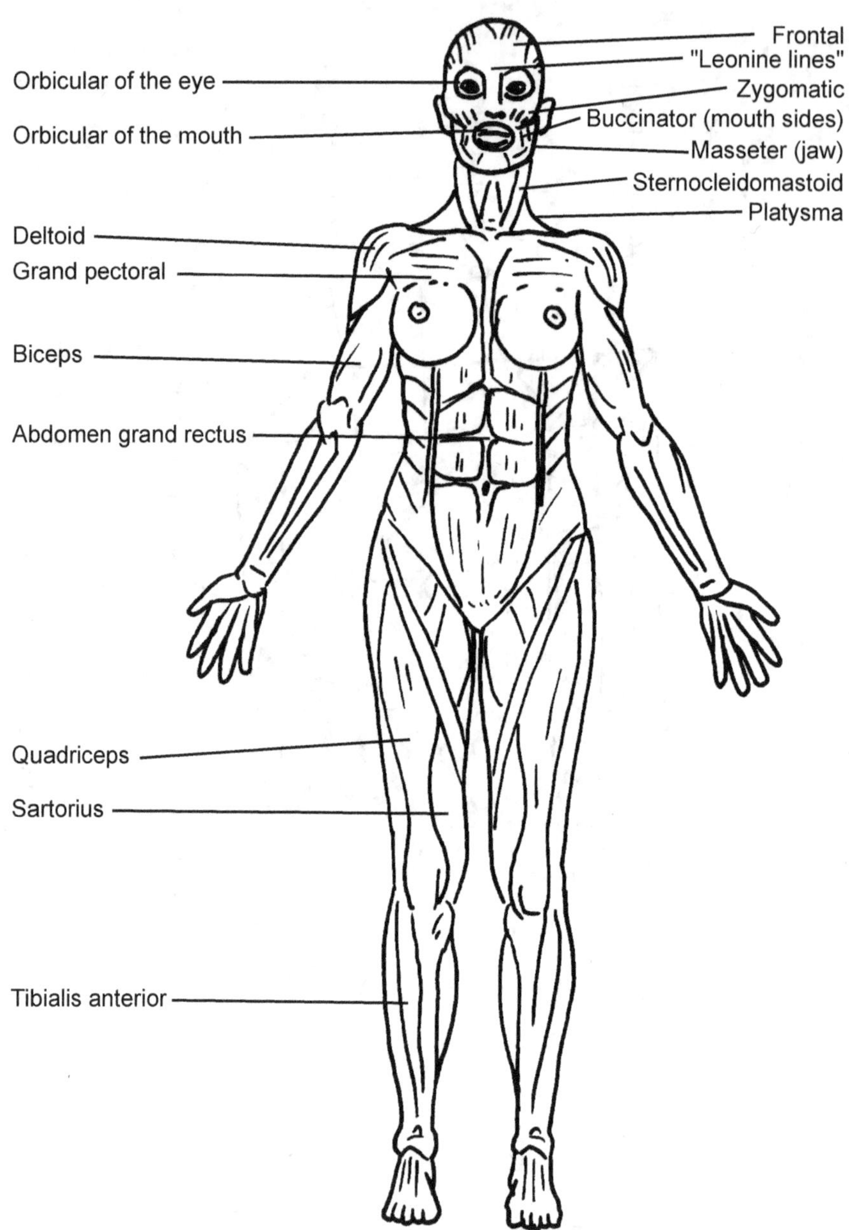

Illustration 2 - Muscular apparatus (front, face and neck)

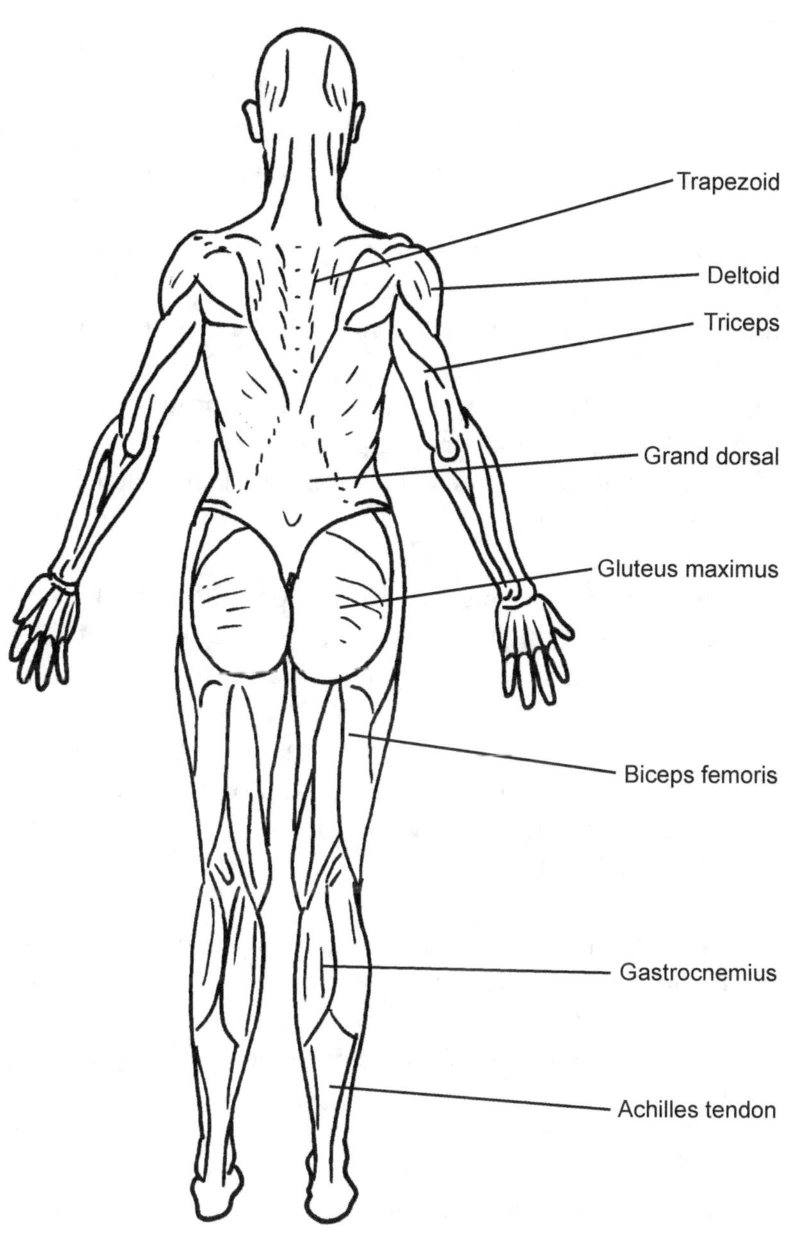

Illustration 3 - Muscular apparatus (rear)

Human anatomy

The skeleton of the human body is formed by around 206 bone pieces, among head, thoracic cage, lower and upper limbs, included the vertebral column, which connects the head to the pelvis.

The bones' function is precious, since, other than to keep us standing, they enclose the internal organs, protecting them.
The skull enclose and protect the brain, fundamental element of all the actions of our life.

The thoracic cage enclose the liver: blood filter; the lungs: blood oxygenators, and the heart: pump for the circulation of the blood which it makes to flow in every vein of our body.

The dorsal spine encloses the spinal marrow which extends up to the pelvis and is the connection between the cerebellum and the nervous system, and it give to the human body the opportunity to stand up and do activities.

The bones are a splendid scaffold, but they couldn't keep us standing or do other activities, if they wouldn't sustained and connected one each other by the tendons and covered by muscular tissues that, other than giving elasticity and movement, they give also a human shape (in our case).

From the bones several muscles take their names, and the muscles give their names to the movement that the beautician must know perfectly and execute it in the right direction to reactivate the functionality and the elasticity needed by the body.

The most important muscles to deal with are:

Rear:

Femoral (thigh)
Gastrocnemius (calf)
Gluteuses (buttocks)
Dorsal (back)
Trapezoid (between the shoulders)
Deltoid (shoulders)
Triceps (arm)

Front:

Tibialis (leg)
Quadriceps (thigh)
Abdomen (stomach)
Pectorals (breast)

Face and neck:

Platysma (neck)
Orbicular of the mouth (lips)
Mentalis square (chin)
Masseter (jaw)
Buccinator (between mouth and cheekbones)
Zygomatic (cheekbones)
Orbicular of the eyes (eyes border)
Temporal (temples)
Frontal (forehead)

All these muscles have a voluntary action, and move mechanically on our command.

But there are muscles with involuntary action that move even without our will, but with the stimulus of the emotion, for example: the heart and the stomach.

End of fourth lesson

Verification questions:

- From where do some muscles' name comes from?
- What do connect head and pelvis?
- How many bones do the human body have?
- Can you tell at least 5 muscles of the body?

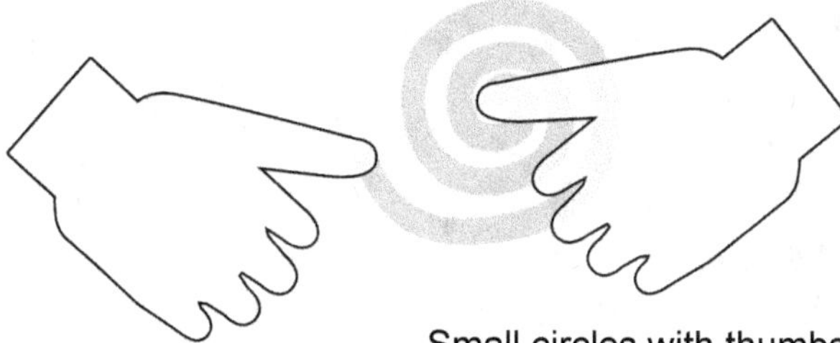

Small circles with thumbs to close the movement

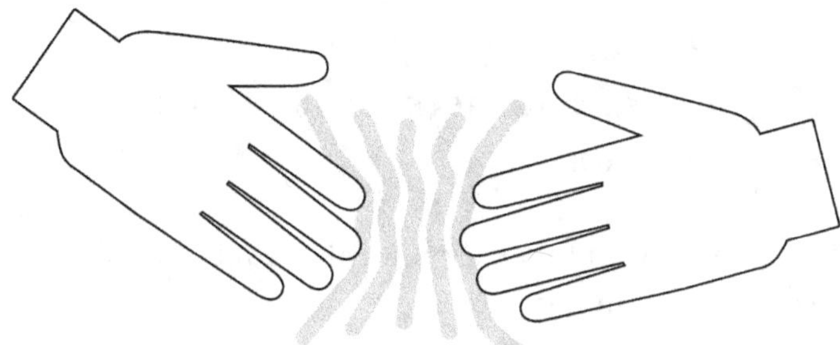

Rubbing with the four fingers on front

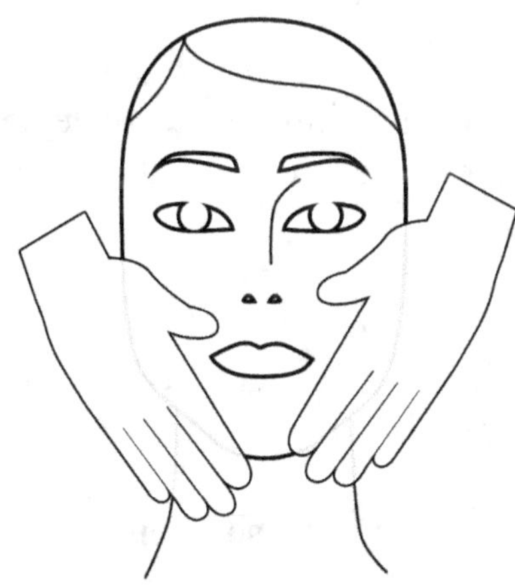

Caressing with open hands

Illustration 4 - Massage movements

What is needed in this lesson:

- A massage cream
- A phial of massage oil, even vegetable

The massage (1)
to pectoral, platysma and sternocleidomastoid muscles

The muscles we are dealing in this lesson, of the front, are of big importance for woman's femininity.

In fact, in these points of the body the ageing arrives soon and can be noticed at first sight for their focal point; thus it is good to prevent it on time.

The pectoral muscle covers the breast, while the sternocleidomastoid starts from the base of the neck and runs up to the ears' rear, the platysma at last covers the whole neck.

The movements to massage the pectoral include the caressing and the rubbing; same for the platysma and the sternocleidomastoid keeping in mind to avoid the pushing of the middle part of the neck (oesophagus).
These movements have to be executed with some pressure, to awake an adequate blood circulation.

Execution of the massage

Standing behind the client who will have the head leaned on the headrest, pass with both hands a little of massage cream on the pectorals and on the neck; this will help the impact and the sliding of the moving hands.

Now with the open hands caress starting from breasts up to the chest, décolleté and the shoulders (deltoid); stop here and with the thumbs do the usual circle to close the movement.

Now restart from décolleté and go up forming many circles with the fingers; alternate these two movements two times each.

Return at the base of the neck, this time with the hands on the front, and press the skin by pinching it between the index and the middle fingers of both hands; then, with both open hands, pass again with a caressing movement; alternate these movements two times for each side.

Remember that it is not much the form of the massage that brings achievements, but your hands are awaking and modelling that part of the body.

End of fifth lesson

Verification questions:

- What are the kind of massages done on the décolleté?
- In which directions is done the massage?
- Where is the sternocleidomastoid located?

The massage (2)
to chin, under chin and masseter (jaw)

These muscles, as their name tells, cover the square of the chin giving it shape and support.

The muscles of this group intersect under the cheekbone with the masseter and the buccinator, like in a really solid web of big importance; because altogether they sustain the lower part of the face, that with ageing usually often to fall, forming that unaesthetic cutaneous relaxation.

This is the reason why chin, under chin, and jaw represent the strong line of the face that have to be activated.

Execution of the massage

Standing behind the client, after having spread the cream, start from the centre of the chin with both hands and caress along the jaw; here with the thumbs do the circle to close the movement.

Repeat, but this time from under the chin to the jaw, alternating over and below quickly for five times closing with the final circle.

Now move at the right side of the client and with the hands in front, press the skin between index and middle fingers pinching, going up along the masseter and buccinator, repeating also to the left side; then with the hands go back again to the chin and again go up along the muscles with caressing movement.

Repeat these movements two times for each side.

End of sixth lesson

Verification questions:

- Which role do the chin muscles have?
- Which massage movements are used in these lesson?
- List the muscles of this lesson.

The massage (3)
to orbicular of the eyes, frontal and nose muscles

The nose is made of a cartilage protuberance and is covered only by skin: its muscles are attached only to its base (pyramidal).

This is so also for the eyelids in which the only muscle (a sphincter) is attached to their edge.

Also in the forehead, even if of bigger size, we find the muscles attached just to the temporal bone (temples), this way leaving all the central forehead skin to move without restraints.

Thus, for either nose, eyes and forehead, the movements of the massage must be done with caution, following the peculiar natural muscular line.

Execution of the massage

Standing behind the client with the hands laid on the base of the nose, start the massage: pulling out the thumbs of both hands, form many small circles going up along the walls of the nose up to his base between the brows; then rub here with the thumbs crossed like an X; all three times.

This last movement is useful to remove those unaesthetic creases (called "leonine"); it is to be repeated two times or more.

Now with the hands laid over the eyes pull out the index and middle fingers of both hands and caress the eyelids stopping at the edges forming the small circle as closing movement; repeat two or three times.

Now pass to the frontal: with the hands at the centre of the forehead, caress up to the temples, stop here and do the usual circle with the hands; then repeat three times trying to put vigour to these movements so that they could stir and warm this part of the face, a bit cold and not much muscular.

Now with the open hands (and in case with a little of cream) restart from the décolleté, neck, jaw and up back along over all the muscles with a "kneading" movement, up to the frontal, mitigating and warming in one only movement all the muscles.

It is important to feel that under the hands the skin is hot and it have absorbed the massage cream, and that the muscles have awaken.

End of seventh lesson

Verification questions:

- Of which tissue is the nose made?
- How can be called the eyelid muscle?
- Where the forehead muscles are attached?

The massage (4)
to orbicular mouth, buccinator and masseter muscles

The muscles of the mouth are called orbicular, for they orbit around the mouth opening, giving it elasticity and support.

The function of the mouth orbicular, like those of the eyes, is very important, because they alone have to sustain that part of the face which is independent from the other, and for this reason it is very prone to the relaxing and the formation of creases and wrinkles.

What said above is valid also for the platysma of the neck, which remains independently alone.

Thus, keeping these muscles in good function we will avoid its premature ageing and the formation of those characteristic vertical creases, like "monkey's lip", as for the sagging eyelids, like "chinese eyes", or the creases of the neck forming rings.

Also the masseter and the buccinator, that are found between the edges of the mouth and the jaw, are a cause of ageing of the face: keeping them in good function with the massage, we will avoid those fatal creases over and under the edges of the mouth, called smile wrinkles the upper ones and sadness wrinkles the lower ones.
These creases are typical in those who smile much or those who are often of sad mood.

Execution of the massage

Standing behind the client, and after having spread the massage cream or oil, put the two hands on the centre of the mouth and open the index and middle fingers of both hands forming a V, then caress the orbicular of the mouth up to the ears, three times, stopping at the edges of the mouth and forming a small circle with the thumbs to close the movement, and pressing a little.

Now with the hands as fists, pull out the thumbs and starting from the chin go up along the masseter and the buccinator forming many small circles (rubbing); then with the index and middle fingers of the two hands caress again the mouth orbicular and then repeat these movements two times each.

These movements must be done always in ascending direction, this is to say always from low to high.

This kind of manual massage is the best, because the hand makes the skin elastic. The movement can be modified from mild to energetic, depending on the need, to obtain a perfect result and to arrive in any part of the body. Anyway we can take advantage (nowadays in particular) also of excellent devices, that relieve the hard work of the operator and they give good results too.

End of eighth lesson

Verification questions:

- Why the mouth muscles are called orbicular?
- How the upper creases of the lip are also called?
- Where the masseter and buccinator muscles are found?

What is needed in this lesson:

- Rose water
- Cream or powder peeling
- A small basin non metallic
- A bristle brush
- Water
- A sponge for removal
- Some cotton wool

The peeling

The peeling is a deep cleaning of the skin because it removes the dead cells of the horny layer, revealing the layer of new cells.

The peeling may be as cream, as powder and as gum, or chemical for a deep action, but the latter is of medical expertise because the skin is being burned by an acid for a total cutaneous renewal.

We will deal of the mild one, as cream or powder.

Today, the easier way is the cream, ready for application as a simple beauty mask and that has the same characteristics of the traditional one which have to be prepared.

Once it was more widespread the gum kind, which is applied hot like a depilatory wax and it is removed cold with tweezers, which is not much practical even if the results are excellent.

Execution

Put an amount of peeling like a chestnut into a non metallic basin, dissolve with some drops of water and pass the paste on all the face with a brush, starting from the décolleté and then up to the face and forehead, keeping lips and eyes clean, since they may get irritations.

Once the application is ended, keep quiet for fifteen minutes, with the eyes covered by a small piece of cotton soaked with water rose, and the head laid on the headrest.

Removal

Take a small beautician sponge, soak it and wet all the treated part removing any trace of the paste with movements from low to top and circular.

Rinse the sponge from time to time avoiding drippings into the eyes. After the removal apply a cloth or a damp sponge to refresh the skin. Then pass the mask which will be the next lesson's topic.

End of ninth lesson

Verification questions:

- What is peeling?
- What is the difference between mild and chemical peeling?
- What are we removing with peeling?

What is needed in this lesson:

- A beauty mask for the skin type we are dealing with
- A small basin
- A brush
- Water
- A small sponge
- Rose water

The mask

The mask is the ideal treatment to end a good work: it is the secret weapon of every beautician; in fact, only after the mask, the client will notice that sensation of freshness and of a more tight and luminous skin.

The mask is this essential after every beauty treatment.

There are many kinds of masks and it is important to choose the appropriate type: as powder, as cream, for oily skins, for dry skins and for skin with acne; you can find them in perfumeries or by hairdressers' wholesale dealers.

How to use

With an already cleansed skin, apply the mask with a clean small brush, after having mixed it into a non metallic basin with some drops of water or some tonic lotion appropriate to the type of skin.

Spread the mask starting from the décolleté and up along the neck, chin, cheeks, nose and forehead, keeping away from eyes in order to avoid dripping it into them and irritations.

Leave it to rest for fifteen minutes with the head laid on the armchair and with cotton wool pieces wet with rose water over the eyelids.

During the rest it is necessary an absolute quiet, because the skin have to avoid the forming of creases due to speaking or smiling, which would compromise the good success of the mask.

Removal

Once the rest time is passed, take a small sponge damp with water, wet all the face and remove all the mask starting from the low to the high, often rinsing the sponge, till there will be no trace of it.

At the end pass a fresh wipe with some drops of tonic lotion. Rose water is essential: very refreshing.

End of tenth lesson

Verification questions:

- When the beauty mask have to be applied?
- With which tool is the mask applied?
- Why is quiet necessary during the rest time?

What is needed in this lesson:

- A tonic lotion appropriate for the skin type
- Some absorbent cotton wool
- A beautician stick or small sponge

The tapping and analysis of the skin

In this lesson we will talk about tapping that, even if brief, we have to emphasize its strong action in removing the torpor in some slack skins taking them to a fresh and active state.

In fact it is not uncommon to see some visages with a weary skin, opaque, flaccid and cold like without life.

This state may have been determined by an illness, a depression: the causes are many, but to know the skin and its characteristics two are the methods: the first is called *Espetio* the second *Palpatio*.

Espetio, which in Greek means "by the appearance", means that looking with naked eye or with the magnifier we can notice the state and its needs.

Palpatio, as it can be argued by the word, means that palpating the skin with the hands, we can feel its grain, its temperature, its tone, the elasticity, its deficiencies and what are its needs.

To analyse the skin in this way it is very important because we will have more expertise for the beauty cares.

The tapping

With the skin already cleansed, take a wet sponge for beauticians and pass it on all the face, starting from the neck, up to the forehead tapping repeatedly till the skin would have got that tonicity it needs.

Repeat if it is the case with another tonic and a sponge afresh.

It is important to use the appropriate tonic for that particular skin type we are dealing with.

Thus, if the skin we are treating is dry, the tonic will be soft, like rose water, fruity, but never alcoholic.
On the contrary, if the skin is oily, it shall be preferable an astringent tonic, thus a little alcoholic.

In the cases of a skin excessively weary and relaxed, we can take advantage of the fingers of the hands tapping with the soft of the fingertips on the whole face: this will give tonicity in an effective and incredible way.

End of eleventh lesson

Verification questions:

- With an oily skin, which tonic have to be used?
- What are the names of the methods to analyse the skin?
- What is the function of the tapping?

Products for the make-up:

- Day cream or beauty milk
- Foundation cream of the proper colour
- Stick for dark circled eyes
- Face powder in powder or solid
- Cheeks blusher
- Eye pencil
- Lips pencil
- Lipstick
- Eyelids blusher
- Big brush for face powder
- Small and thin brush the eye line

The basic make-up

The make-up is the secret weapon of the woman: it is the art of transformation to appear more beautiful; the beautician is its master par excellence, because he have the secrets of know how.

Nowadays the make-up is become almost a custom, as it happens in all the tribes (the American Natives for examples); so the women have got it as a common habit to be more pleasant.

Make-up means to have a better appearance not letting the other to notice that the make-up has been done.

We can do even much catchy make-ups, as, for example, for the theatre or in the movies, or to mask oneself.

The important thing in the make-up is to turn evident the positive aspects of a face, hiding the defects.

The colours to realize it must be matching with the colours of the hair and the eyes, so that the lines would appear mitigated and not exaggerated.

Tones for the types: blonde, chestnut and red:

Foundation creams:	all the golden or amber beiges.
Pencils:	chestnut, brown.
Eye shadows:	azure, bright blue, sage, violet.
Lips:	rose, cyclamen, geranium.
Conccalcrs:	Sienna earth, bronze, beige.
Face powders:	beige, golden, umber.

Tones for the types: brown, dark chestnut, grey:

Foundation creams:	pearl or golden beiges.
Pencils:	brown, grey, blue.
Eye shadows:	grey, blue, azure, violet.
Lips:	bright red, orange, geranium.
Concealers:	Sienna earth, dark, cheek red, beige.
Face powders:	pearl, golden or umber beiges.

To do a make-up to a regular face it is better to follow one's own features; but if the eyes, the mouth or the brows are a little sagging, with the pencils try to raise them toward the edges.
For close eyes and brows, pluck the brows in the centre and lengthen

toward the temples with the pencil.

If the mouth is too small, with thin lips, pass the pencil a bit on the outer edge of the lips then fill the inside with the lipstick. If otherwise it is too wide, do the contrary: pass the pencil with a darker tone than lips, on the inner edge and the fill with the lipstick.

To correct recessed cheeks, dark circled eyes or skin stains, we have to use bright concealers, as paste or stick.

To to make a face slim or to mitigate a bony edge, we have to use a dark and coating concealer in the point we want to make it to disappear. Then pass the foundation appropriate to the chosen colour.

To correct a face it is also important a proper hair style.

Execution

After having cleansed the skin of neck and face, spread with the small sponge or with the hands a bit of beauty cream or milk; in the same way spread evenly the foundation cream, then some bright stick on the eye sockets and some blusher on the cheeks fading with the fingers; then pass the face powder on the whole face and neck with cotton wool. A mildly wet napkin barely laid on the skin of the visage will fix the make-up.

On the upper eyelids pass some shadow, fading it; then a light line of pencil on the edge of the eyes and on the brows.

At last a light line of pencil on the mouth borders and then the lipstick.

It is good to remind that the colours of the make-up are prone to the trend variations, thus we will utilize also the colours of that time, keeping always in mind the basic knowledge.

There is not a make-up suitable for everybody, but one makes the visage up depending the needs, even a little may be sufficient. The most important thing is the skin type, a good coating foundation and everything will be perfect.

End of twelfth lesson

Verification questions:

- What do make-up means?
- How to resize a too wide mouth?
- How to correct a very recessed face?
- If a face is regular, how to make it up?

Mary

Mary, whose registered name is Mariucci Maria, was born in Cortona (Arezzo), Italy.

She qualified as Beautician in 1958 in Turin, under the guide of the great and notorious teacher A. Melis from Istituto Anglem.
For 20 years she has been devoted to this Beautician and Hair Stylist work, from Perugia to Genua, working and teaching.

Then she became devoted to writing and drawing, and she directed television programs of Cosmetics. In the 80s the Italian magazine Bella published for her a report, which gave her the chance to correspond with women readers, giving solutions and cosmetics advices.

Having skills of make-up drawing, she always had an interest and admiration for art, so since when she retired she devoted also to painting; check the following website where it is possible to know his Naïve Art of Primitive mark and also to contact her in person.

It is a big love for aesthetics, and art in general, which Mary wants to hand down to the posterity.

Contacts

Mary - Art Naïve, Art Brut, Primitive Art, Raw Art
http://jizaino.cf/mary

ringthebell@libero.it